About this book

This book will give you the facts about braces—what they're like, why you need them, and how they work. You'll find out what to expect and what you can do to make your treatment go smoothly and quickly. You'll find out the answers to the following questions and many more:

• What is orthodontics?

• What is a bad bite?

• What can I expect from orthodontic treatment?

• When is the right time for braces?

• What kind of treatment will I need?

• How do braces work?

Remember—the information in this book is general. You are a unique individual. Your own dentist's advice is the best advice you can get.

COASTAL CONSUMER HEALTH LIBRARY
New Hanover Regional Medical Center

What is orthodontics?

Orthodontics is a special type of dentistry that deals with the correction of *bad bites*, or problems with the way your teeth fit together. Many dentists have been trained to provide orthodontic treatment. For more complex cases, an orthodontist, a specially trained dentist who does orthodontic treatment only, can provide care.

No matter who does your treatment, a visit to your family dentist is always the first step.

What's so bad about a bad bite?

Imagine two saw blades that come together in a perfect match like pieces of a puzzle. This is how your upper and lower teeth should fit together when you close your mouth.

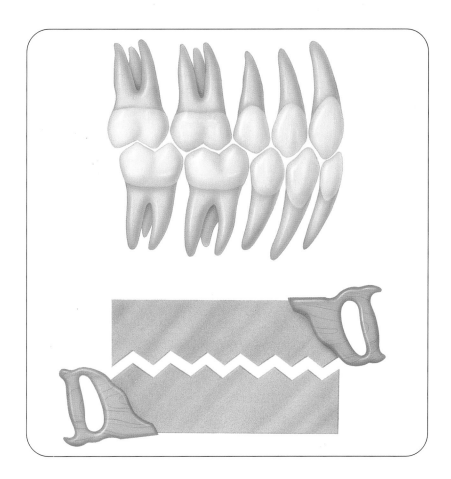

If your teeth don't fit together like this, you have a bad bite (or *malocclusion*).

Having a bad bite affects more than just the way you look. It may make it difficult for you to speak, swallow, and chew, and it may cause unnecessary wear to your teeth.

A bad bite may make it harder to clean your teeth and mouth thoroughly, which could cause cavities, gum disease, and bad breath.

About your teeth

To understand why you have a bad bite, it helps to know a little bit about teeth and how they develop.

The teeth are firmly anchored in the bone of the upper and lower jaws. Underneath the gums, the bottom part of the tooth, called the *root*, holds the tooth within the bone, with the help of fibers, or *ligaments*. The top part of the tooth, called the *crown*, is what we can see.

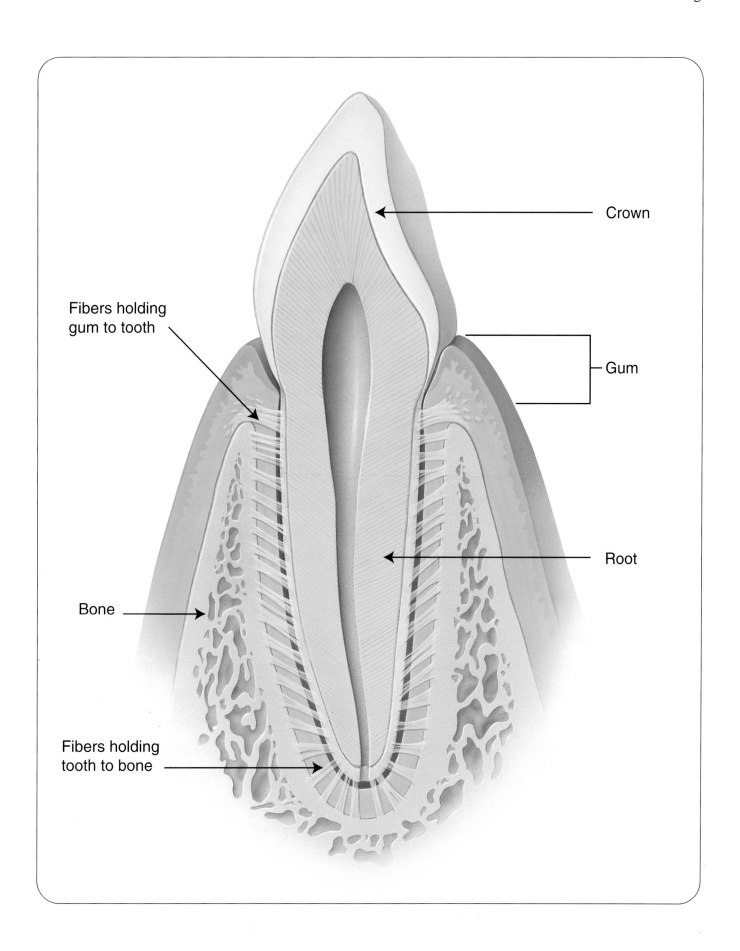

Crown

Fibers holding
gum to tooth

Gum

Root

Bone

Fibers holding
tooth to bone

How the bite develops

The bones in your face go through many changes as you grow. Even though teeth may look and feel like bones, they don't behave in the same way. Bones continue to develop for as long as you are growing, but crowns are full size even before they grow out of the gums, or *erupt*, into the mouth.

The front teeth and molars (shown in blue) are the first permanent teeth to erupt. They leave space between them for the remaining permanent teeth. If the teeth don't fit into the space exactly, a bad bite may result.

From the time the permanent teeth begin to develop in the jaw until they replace the baby teeth, many different forces work together to form the bite. These include the growing jaw bones, and all the different muscles used to cry, suck, swallow, breathe, and speak.

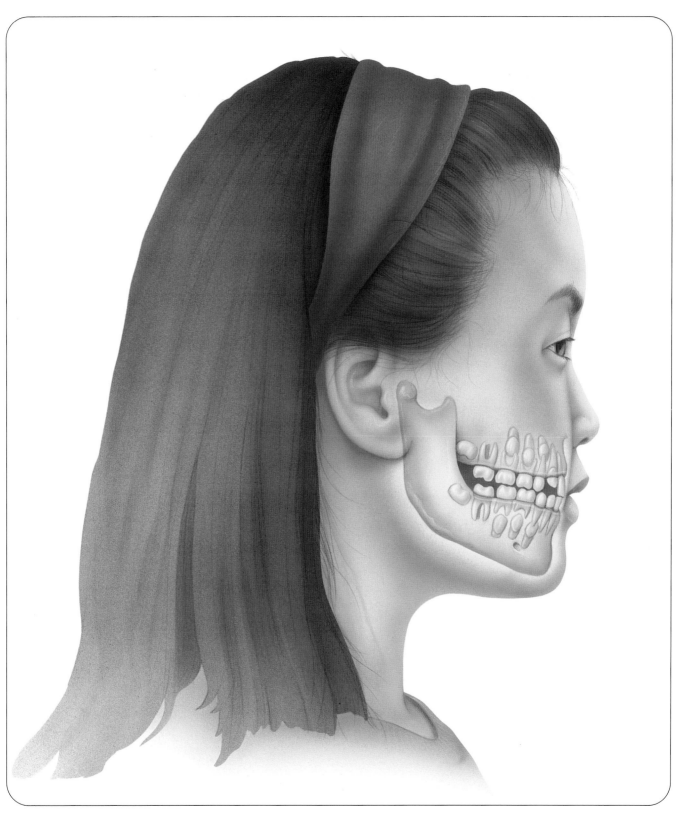

This girl still has some of her baby teeth (shown in pink). Her front teeth and first molars have grown in, but not all of her permanent teeth (shown in blue) have erupted.

What is a bad bite?

In an ideal bite, the front teeth overlap slightly, and the edges of your lower teeth should touch the inner surfaces of the upper teeth.

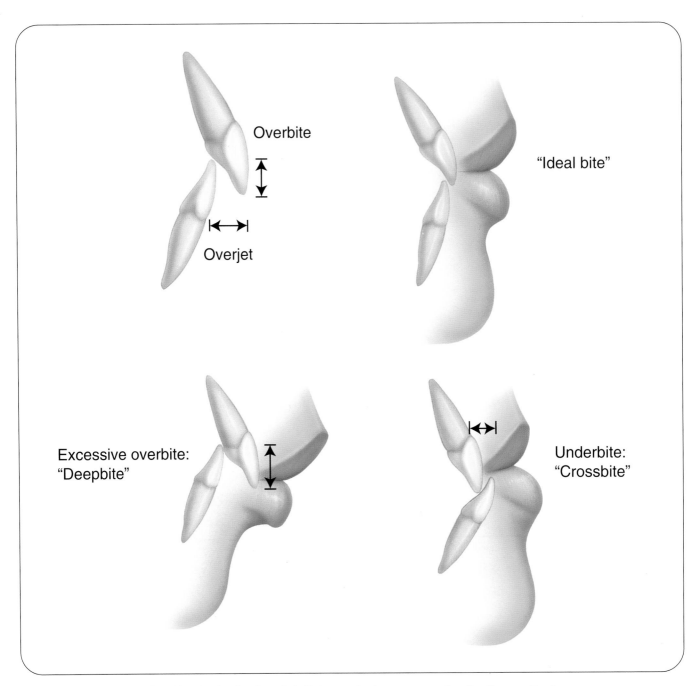

Overbite

Overjet

"Ideal bite"

Excessive overbite: "Deepbite"

Underbite: "Crossbite"

Overjet is the horizontal distance between your teeth; the vertical distance is called overbite.

If the front teeth come down too far, it's called a "*deepbite*." A "*crossbite*" can happen when the size of your lower jaw does not match the size of your upper jaw, and some of your bottom teeth are on the outsides of your top teeth when you bite down.

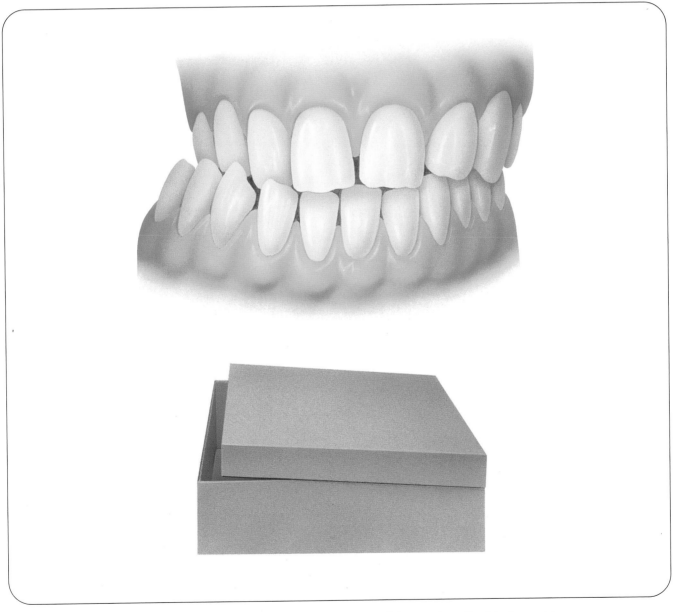

A crossbite is similar to trying to fit a lid on a box that is too wide or long for it—no matter how you try, one side of the lid always ends up inside the box.

What type of bad bite do I have?

There are many different types of bad bites. Most problems can be grouped into one of three major classifications, based on how the first molars (shown in blue) meet each other when the mouth is closed. This system is called Angle's Classification, after the early American orthodontist, Edward H. Angle.

Remember, each bad bite is different. Your problem may not fit into any single group.

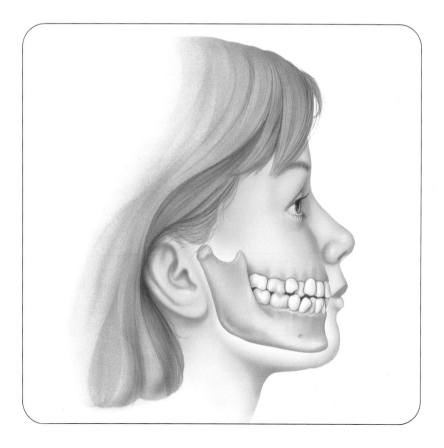

Class I: The jaws are in the correct position, but the teeth are crooked.

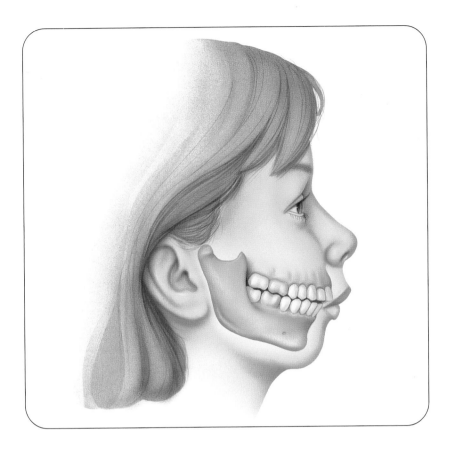

Class II: The upper jaw juts out too far, which results in "buck teeth."

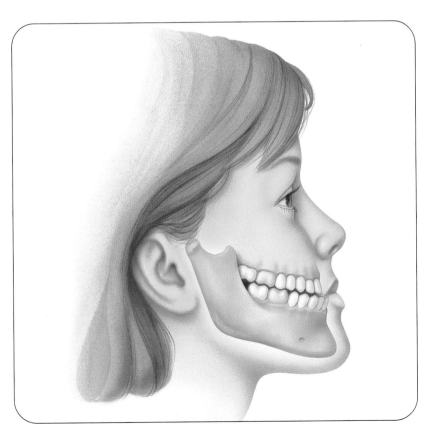

Class III: The lower jaw has outgrown the upper jaw, causing an underbite.

Why are my teeth crooked?

There are many possible explanations for your crooked teeth. Here are the most common ones:

- *Your teeth didn't come in on schedule*

    Most people's teeth grow into the mouth according to a specific timetable. Sometimes the teeth do not erupt in the proper order. Permanent teeth that arrive too early may take up space that later teeth need. Permanent teeth that arrive too late may not have anywhere to go.

- *There's not enough room in your jaws*

    If the space left for your permanent teeth by the developing jaw and the baby teeth is too small, some teeth may be blocked out. The illustration on page 7 shows how the permanent teeth grow in and leave a certain amount of space for the remaining teeth. If this space is too small, teeth will force themselves out even if they have to twist, tip, or come in at strange angles. On the other hand, if the space is too large, there may be gaps between the teeth.

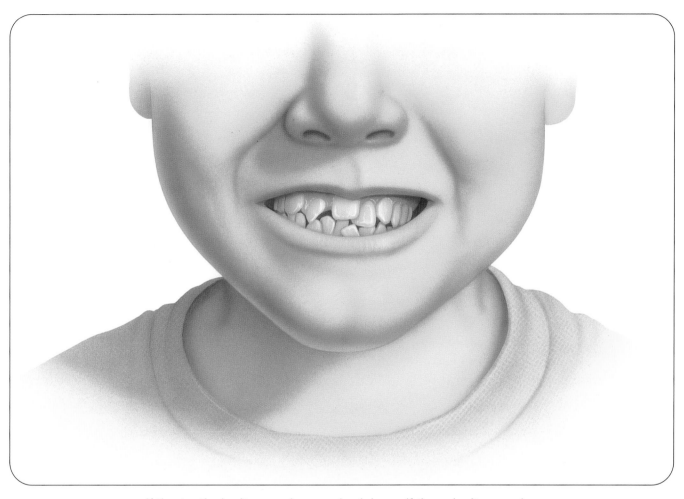

If the teeth don't come in on schedule, or if there isn't enough room in your jaw, you may have crooked teeth.

- *You have extra teeth*

  Extra teeth can take up space, causing the other teeth to crowd.

- *Your molars are in the wrong positions*

  Teeth have tips (*cusps*), with valleys in between them (remember the saw blades?). The cusps of a lower tooth should fit into the valley of the upper tooth. Like the teeth in a broken zipper, if the cusps and valleys of the very first molars do not meet, then all the teeth that come after them will not mesh either. Sometimes, a molar can be so far out of position that its tips meet the valleys of the wrong molar.

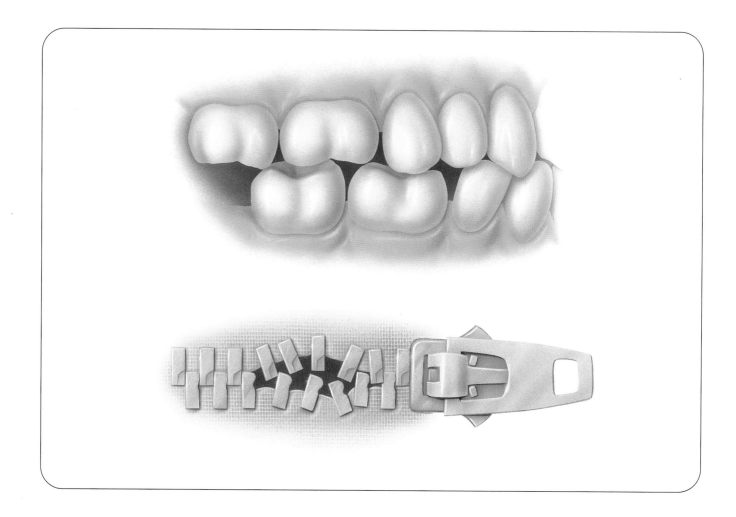

- *You are missing some teeth*

  Sometimes teeth simply don't develop. If this happens, there is too much space, and new teeth may drift into the extra space.

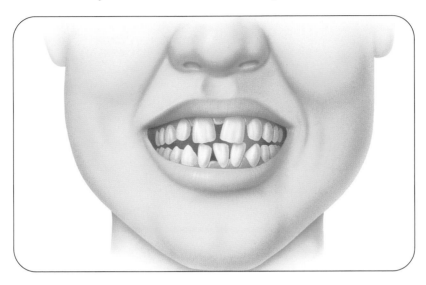

- *Your teeth are too big or too small for your jaw*

  Permanent teeth may be too large or too small for the jaw bone. For example, if you inherited a small jaw from your mother and large teeth from your father, all of your teeth may not fit in your jaw. Also, if a tooth is the wrong size, its tips won't match the valleys of the tooth on the opposite jaw. This child's teeth are too small for the jaw.

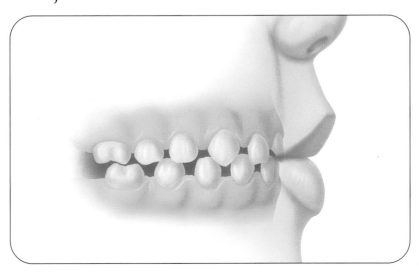

- *You may have had a bad habit*

Sucking your thumb can push your top teeth out and your bottom teeth in, as in the boy shown here. Breathing through your mouth, or pressing your tongue against your front teeth (*tongue thrust*) pushes both your top and bottom teeth apart (shown in box). Both habits can cause an *open bite*.

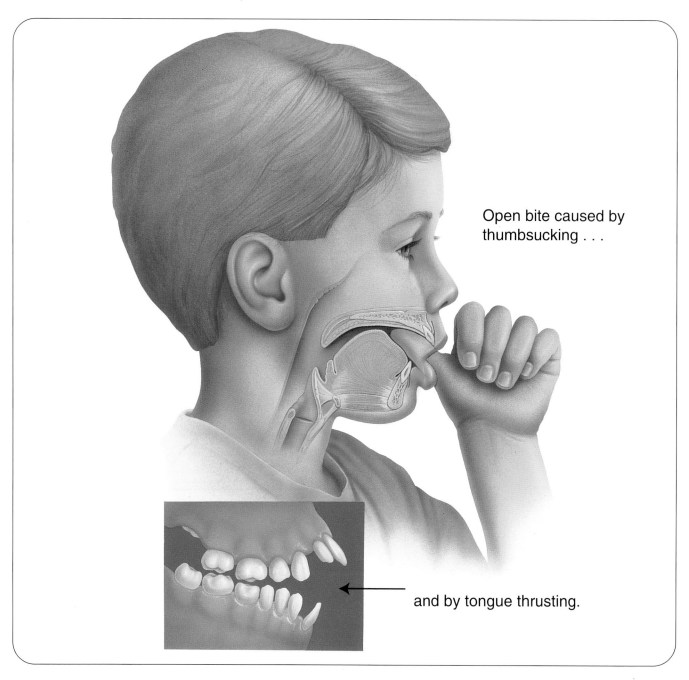

Open bite caused by thumbsucking . . .

and by tongue thrusting.

- *You lost a tooth accidentally*

  Injuries to your face can change how your jaw grows, and cause teeth to be crooked. Chipping your teeth or losing them accidentally will also affect the way your jaw and the rest of your teeth grow.

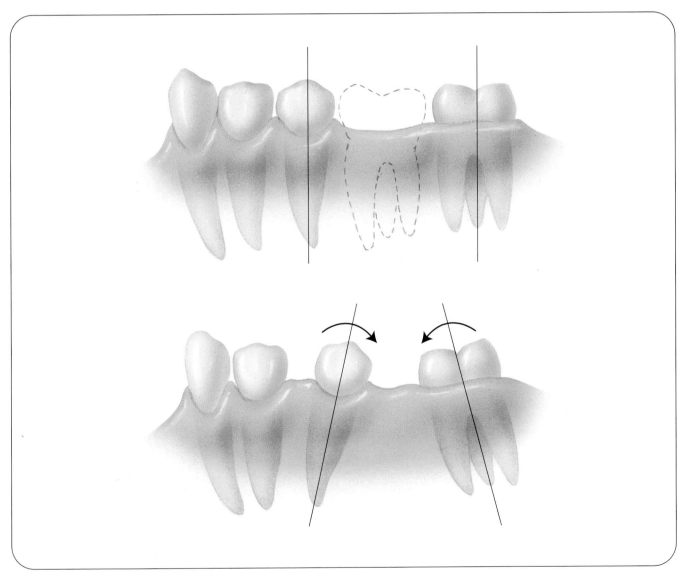

Tooth tipping caused by a missing molar.

When is the right time for braces?

There is no "right age" for braces, and most bad bites can be corrected no matter how old the patient is. The right time for braces is best determined by your dentist. Most people who have orthodontic treatment are younger than 20 years old, but people of all ages can have their teeth straightened.

A common age for an orthodontic examination would be 6 or 7 years, when the first permanent teeth are coming in. Another good time for an orthodontic examination is at age 10 to 12, just before all of the permanent teeth have erupted. Some children with dental developmental problems have orthodontic examinations when they are as young as 2 to 3 years old.

Sometimes, children can be treated at 8 to 10 years of age, and they may not need braces later on. Dentists may place braces on younger patients, which may shorten and simplify treatment later on (*interceptive treatment*).

What can I expect from orthodontic treatment?

The first thing the dentist will probably want to do is examine your teeth, jaw, and face. If you have a bad bite, the dentist or orthodontist will need to study your bite more closely.

To do this, different views of your teeth, jaws, and head will be necessary. This usually involves taking photos of your teeth and face, X-rays of your teeth and head, and making models of your teeth. All of these procedures are painless.

A closer look at your mouth

You will probably be asked to bite down on a soft material to make an *impression*. The dentist will then pour plaster into this impression to make an exact replica of your bite.

This *plaster model* (shown below) will become an important tool for the dentist because it is a record of where your teeth were before the treatment started.

Photographs of your teeth, face, and profile also help the dentist plan your treatment and check your progress.

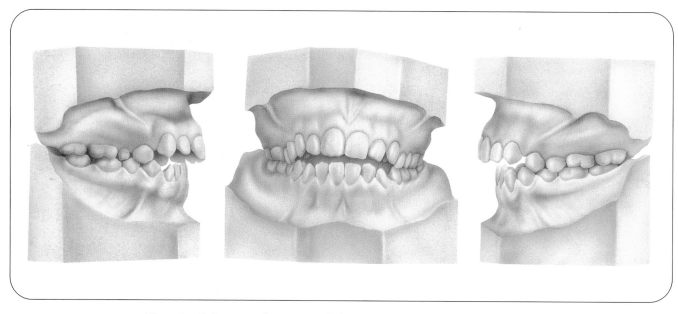

The dentist uses plaster models to plan your treatment and to check the progress of your tooth movement while you have braces.

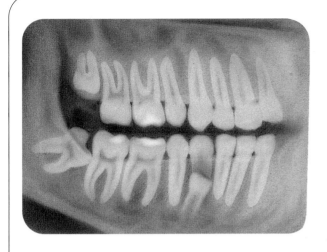

X-rays show the dentist whether you have any cavities, missing teeth, or problems with the roots and bones. The X-ray of the head reveals any problems with the way your teeth or the bones of the upper and lower jaws have developed.

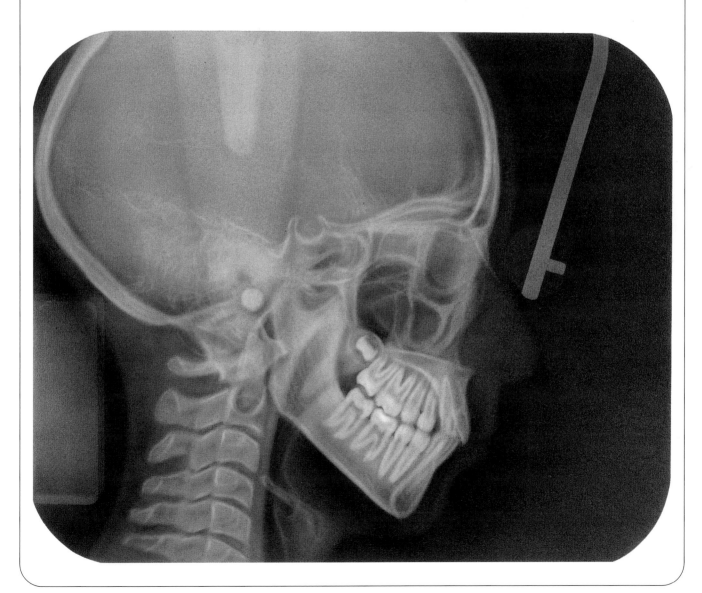

Treatment plan

The dentist will use all of these tools to develop a treatment plan that is just right for your type of bad bite. It is important that you find out exactly what your dentist hopes to achieve with the braces, that is, how your teeth will work and look at the end of the treatment.

You should also find out about how long treatment will last. Remember, this is only an estimate. Many things can lengthen the treatment, but there are some things that may shorten it—including your cooperation, for example, brushing your teeth, keeping a healthy diet, avoiding certain foods, and following the dentist's instructions carefully.

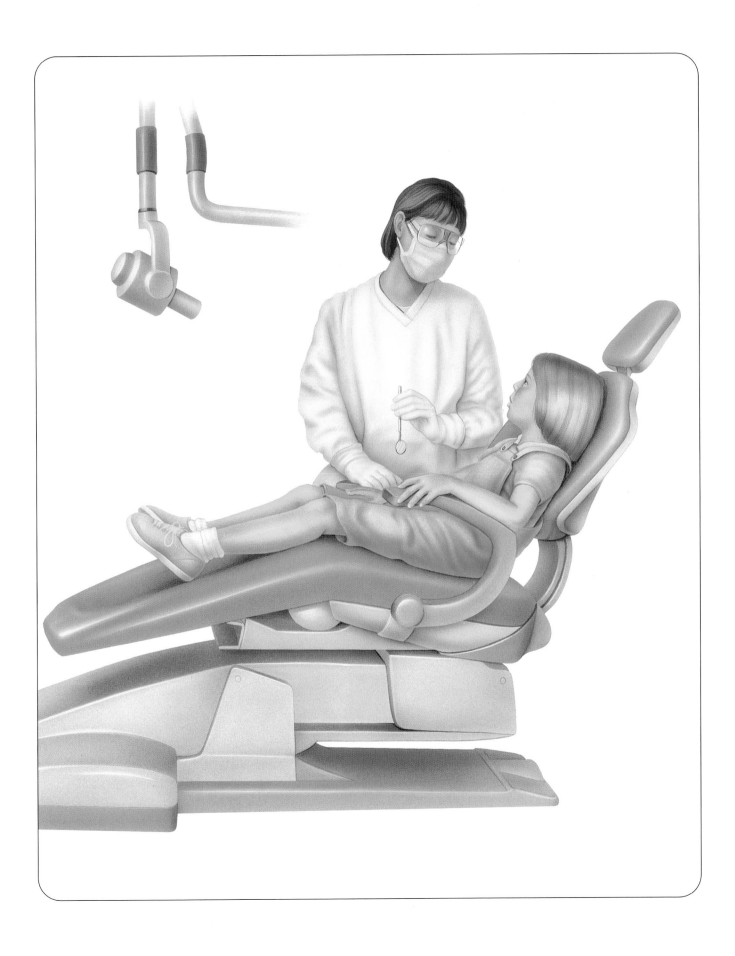

What kinds of braces will I need?

Your dentist will choose the best type of *appliance* to treat your specific problem. The type of treatment depends on whether your teeth or your jaw—or both—need to be fixed.

If your bad bite is caused by problems with the position of your teeth in your jaw, the dentist will probably use braces to straighten them.

Making room for your braces

Sometimes, if your teeth are very close together, the dentist may need to create space between your teeth so that your braces will fit. To do this the dentist uses *separators*, or *spacers*, which are made out of metal or rubber.

Spacers may be uncomfortable for a few days while your teeth are adjusting to them. Children's pain relievers often help.

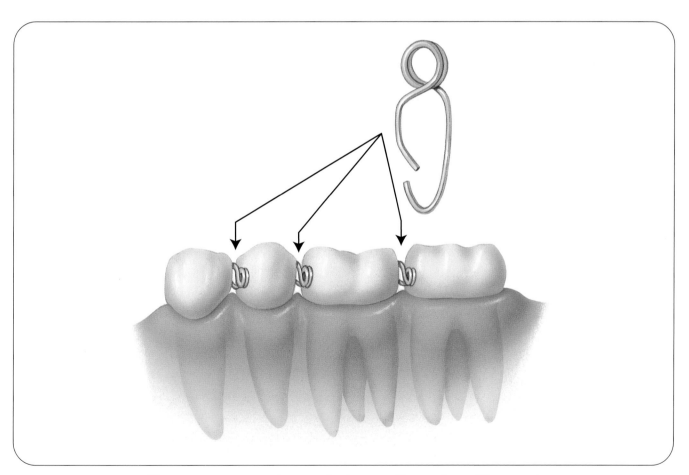

These spacers, made out of wire, act like springs. They push teeth apart to create just enough room for the bands of your braces.

The parts of your braces

The most visible parts of your braces are the square metal *brackets*. These are usually glued directly to your teeth. Like railroad ties that keep the train track in place, the brackets hold the main wire (called the *archwire*) in place. Smaller wires or tiny elastic bands fasten the archwire to the bracket.

If the brackets are not cemented directly to your teeth, they may be attached to a metal *band* that fits around your tooth like a belt. You will most likely have bands around your back molars.

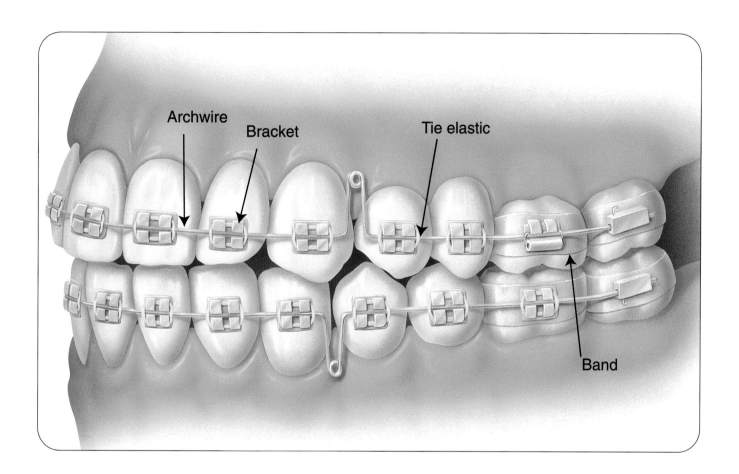

Once these appliances are in place, the dentist may add rubber bands, or additional, smaller wires to put pressure on individual teeth. If you do have rubber bands, you will remove and replace them yourself. Your dentist will show you how to do this and give you a supply of rubber bands.

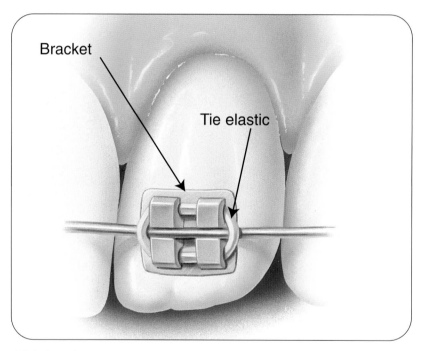

This bracket is bonded to the tooth, and the archwire is held in place by the blue elastic.

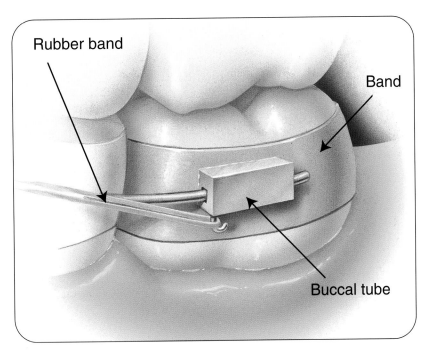

The brackets fastened to the bands on your molar are different from the other brackets. This bracket has a hook for rubber bands.

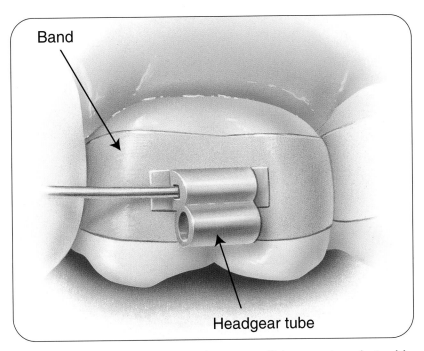

If you have headgear, your braces will have a bracket with a special headgear tube where you will attach the headgear.

30

How braces work

Braces work by applying steady pressure to the teeth, moving them gently and gradually into new positions. This is possible because bone—even though it feels hard, like ivory—is actually flexible. When a tooth is pushed in a certain direction, the bone in front of it gives way under the pressure, and new bone forms behind it to fill the gap.

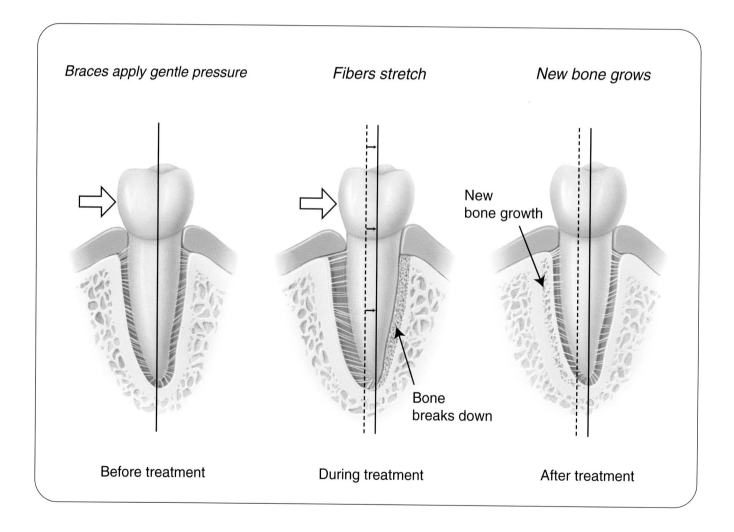

Braces apply gentle pressure   *Fibers stretch*   *New bone grows*

New
bone growth

Bone
breaks down

Before treatment   During treatment   After treatment

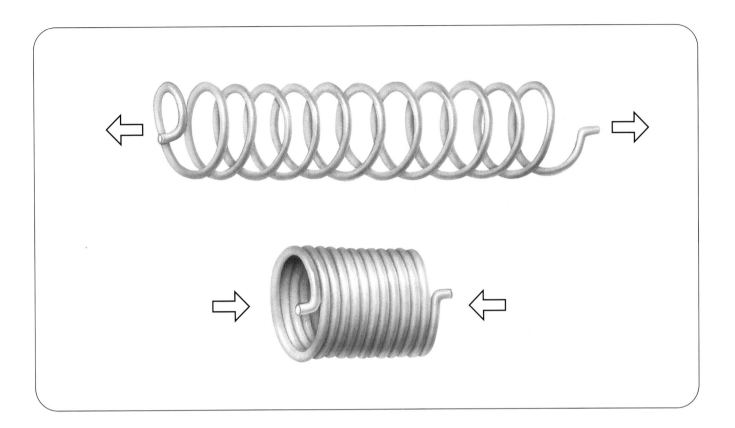

Each wire or rubber band in your braces works like a spring—if you stretch it out and let it go, it returns to its original position. The dentist takes advantage of these forces to move your teeth. The wires or rubber bands are stretched, and as they return to their original positions, they put steady pressure on your teeth, causing them to move.

Problems with the teeth

For a good bite, the upper and lower jaws should have the same number of teeth. If you're missing a tooth because one just didn't grow in, or if you lost one in an accident, the dentist can make a replacement tooth. The replacement tooth is attached to a *retainer*, a removable plastic and wire device that fits into the roof of your mouth. This way, the teeth next to the missing tooth can't drift over into the empty space.

Sometimes, a tooth may be too small compared to the rest of the teeth. This happens most often in the teeth next to the front teeth, the lateral incisors. The dentist can use a special type of plastic to mold a "new" tooth (called a *buildup* or a *crown*) around the one that is too small—and no one can see the difference. This procedure is known as *bonding*. This not only looks better, but it also keeps the neighboring teeth in the right places.

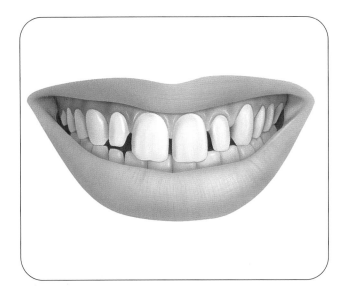

Before bonding

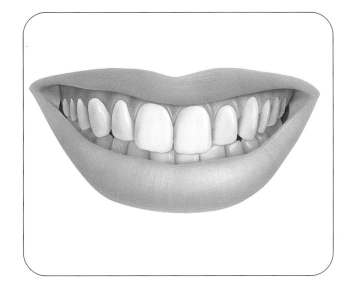

After bonding

Problems with the jaws

Having a bad bite doesn't automatically mean that there's something wrong with your teeth.

Think of a machine with gears that would mesh together correctly, but are mounted in the wrong places. They can't turn, and the machine doesn't work. The situation is the same in your mouth— your teeth may be perfectly sized and positioned, but a problem with your jaws may prevent them from working properly.

The dentist can use different types of appliances to try to control the growth of your jaw.

Helpers for your braces

Any appliance that you wear outside of your mouth is called an *extraoral appliance*; one of the most common ones is called *headgear*. Some people call headgear a "night brace," because it is commonly worn at night while you are sleeping. Headgear usually attaches to the bands around your molars.

There are many different kinds of headgear, but they all use outside forces to help your braces move your teeth. Some have straps that wrap around the top and back of your head (*high pull*), and others have a neck strap (*cervical*).

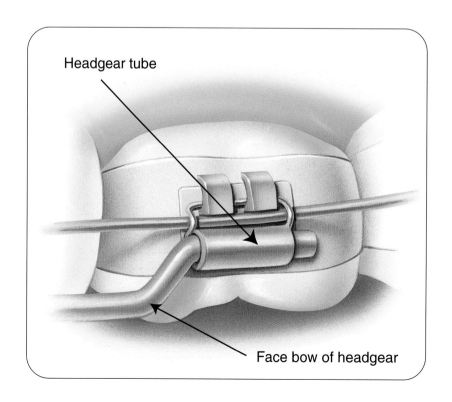

Headgear tube

Face bow of headgear

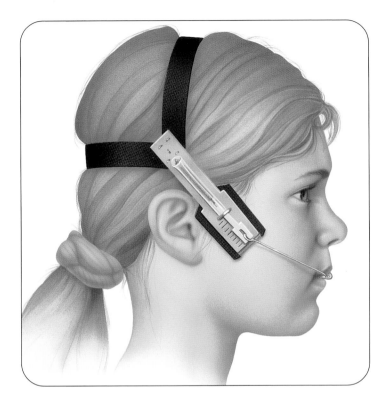

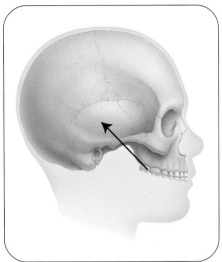

High pull headgear can be used to pull the teeth up and back, or to restrain growth.

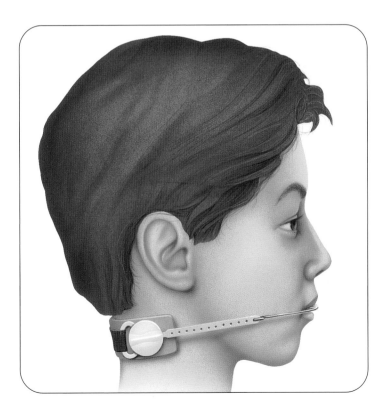

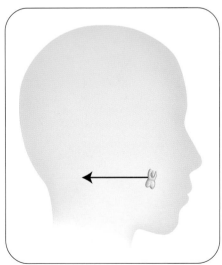

Cervical headgear can be used to help pull the teeth back or to restrain the growth of the upper jaw.

Other appliances

Other appliances that you may have to wear outside of your mouth include *face masks* and *chin cups*.

If your upper jaw is not growing as fast as your lower jaw, a face mask (shown here) can apply gentle pressure to your forehead and chin and even out the rate of growth.

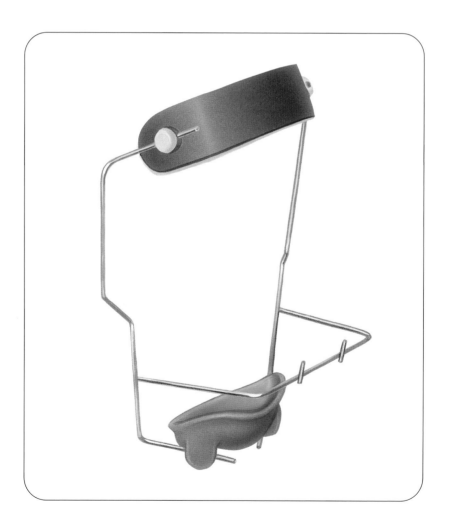

If your lower jaw is too long, the dentist may ask you to wear a *chin cup* to limit your jaw's growth. The chin cup fits around your chin like the chin-strap on a football helmet. It gently pulls the chin upward and backward, slowing its growth.

It is especially important to follow the dentist's instructions. Remember, the more you wear your appliance, the better it works.

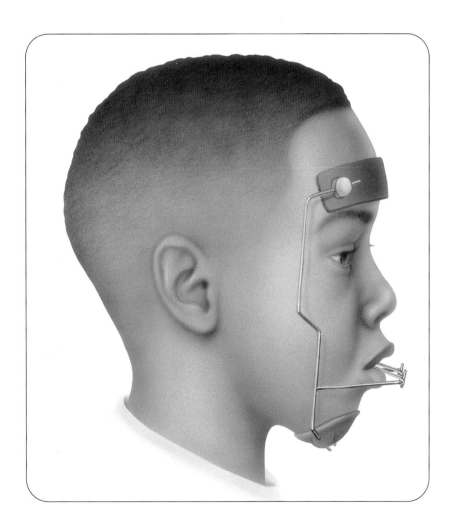

Widening a narrow upper jaw

Even if your teeth are fine, your jaw may still be too narrow, causing you to have a bad bite.

Your dentist may use an *expansion appliance* to widen the roof of your mouth. This works by gradually pushing your upper teeth away from each other. As this happens, new bone forms in the roof of your mouth, making your upper jaw wider.

The new bone normally takes about 1 to 2 months to form, and the upper jaw has to be held in the widened position for 3 to 5 months.

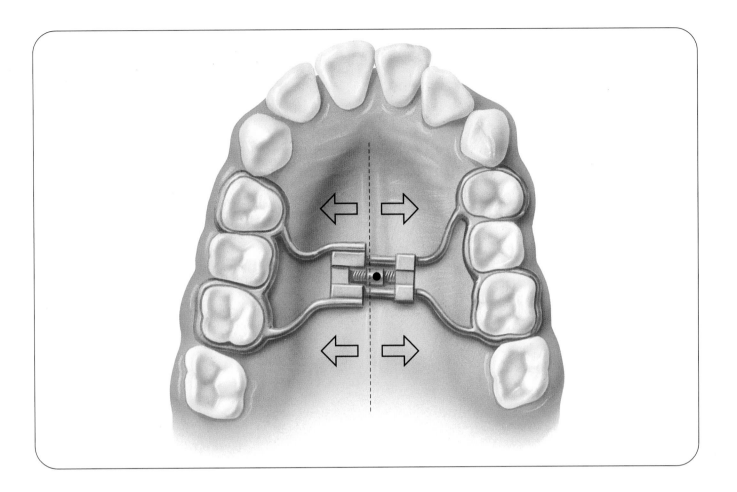

An expansion appliance usually fits into the roof of your mouth like a retainer. It is attached to the teeth on the sides of your mouth. By gently adjusting the width of the appliance, the dentist can gradually push the sides of your upper jaw further apart.

This procedure works best in children from 7 to 15 years old, who are growing anyway.

Correcting a habit or bad bite

Functional appliances work with the natural forces of your muscles to try to influence the way your jaw grows or correct specific problems. They are used to correct a wide range of problems, and can be worn before, after, or with braces.

For example, if you have a habit that affects the way your teeth or jaws are growing, the dentist can design a *habit corrector* that will remind you not to suck your thumb or bite your lip.

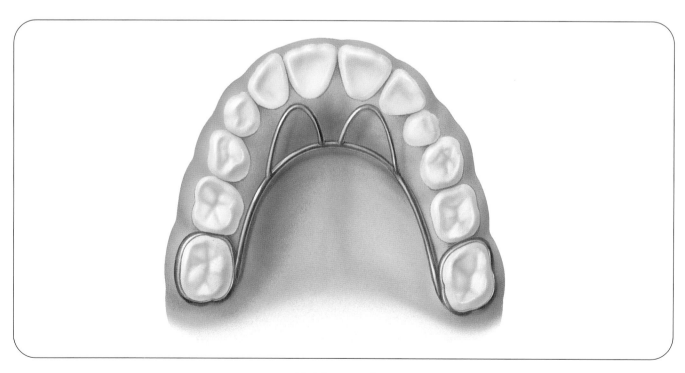

Habit corrector

The dentist may give you a device to wear (when you're not eating) that guides your teeth when you bite down, keeping your jaws in the correct position.

Even though functional appliances can correct a wide range of problems, some bad bites can be fixed only by surgery. For most people, however, the results of treatment with braces and surgery are remarkable.

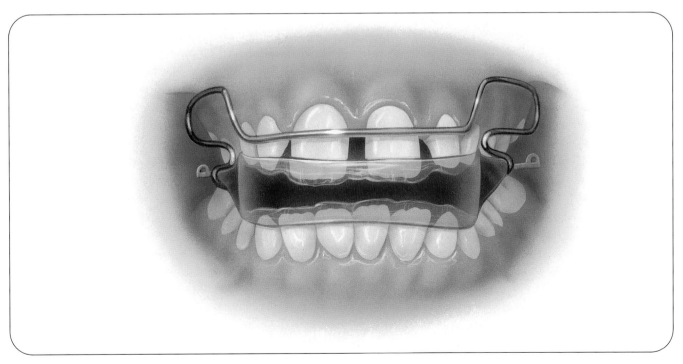

Bite corrector

After you get your braces

Keeping your appointments

One of the most important parts of having braces is making sure that you see your dentist or orthodontist regularly. These appointments are not just check-ups; the adjustments are an essential part of your treatment.

Brushing and flossing

If you look at your braces closely, you will see a tiny ledge where the metal meets your tooth. This space may look really small to you, but to cavity-causing bacteria, it's bigger than the Grand Canyon. It's the most difficult place to clean.

Your dentist will discuss exactly how you should brush and floss, but here are a few tips:

• Come up with a system for covering all sides of all teeth, for example, start with the molars on the top left and work your way through your mouth to the molars on the bottom right. Whichever way you choose, try to stick to your system, and be sure not to forget your back teeth.

• Check your teeth in the mirror to see if you still have any bits of food stuck in your braces.

Cleaning your teeth will be a little more difficult than it was without braces. But with some practice, taking good care of your teeth will become second nature.

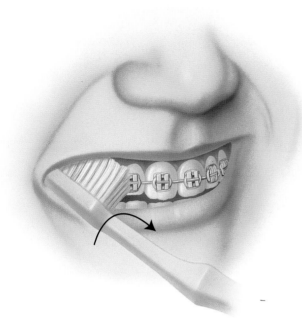

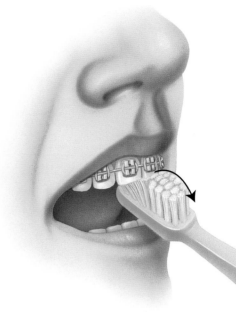

Start with your toothbrush angled against your teeth, making sure you cover the gumline. With a wiping motion, brush the outsides of your teeth, rolling the bristles down and away from them. (Stroke down for your upper teeth and up for your lower teeth.)

For the insides of your teeth, use the tip of your brush.

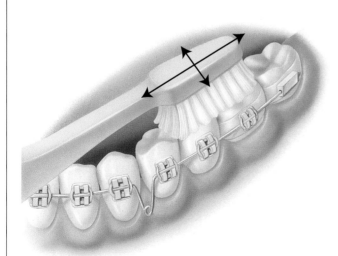

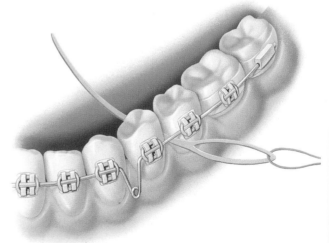

Use the flat surface of your brush to clean the tops of your teeth. Then rinse.

Flossing is more challenging because of the archwire. Your dentist can show you how to floss using a device called a floss threader. This allows you to pass the floss underneath the archwire.

Taking care of your appliances

Your life won't change very much, but you will have to make a few small sacrifices for your straight, healthy teeth.

If you have a removable appliance, be sure to keep it in its protective case when you're not wearing it. If you wrap it in paper towels or tissue, it could easily be mistaken for a piece of trash and get thrown away.

Why can't I...
eat popcorn? Hard foods like popcorn, nuts, corn chips, and ice cubes can damage or break parts of your braces. You can eat some crunchy foods, like apples and carrots, if you cut them into small pieces first. Corn should be cut off the cob.

chew gum? Sticky foods and gum (sugarless gum too) can get caught in braces and loosen them.

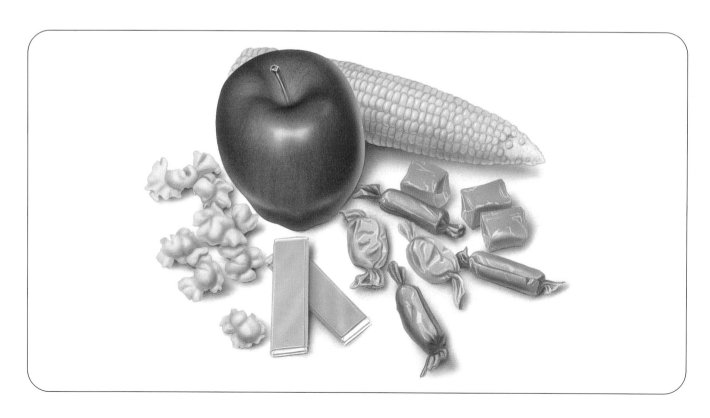

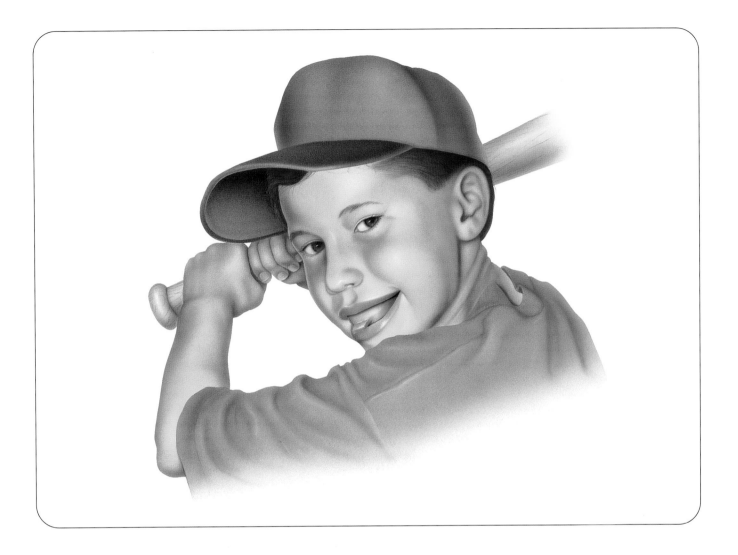

play sports? You can! It's always a good idea—with braces or without—to wear a mouthguard when playing any kind of contact sport.

What if something breaks?

See your dentist immediately, or at least call the office for an appointment and tell them what has happened. If a wire has come loose and is poking you in the mouth, try to gently bend it back into place without breaking it. If this doesn't work, you can put a piece of wax over it until you go to the dentist.

Keeping your teeth in place

After you get your braces off, you will most likely have to wear a retainer to make sure your teeth stay in their new positions long enough for the new bone to harden.

You can take the retainer out when you eat, and to brush and floss. It is important that you wear your retainer as much as possible and that you take good care of it. You should brush your retainer whenever you brush your teeth.

Your dentist will decide how long you will need to wear your retainer.

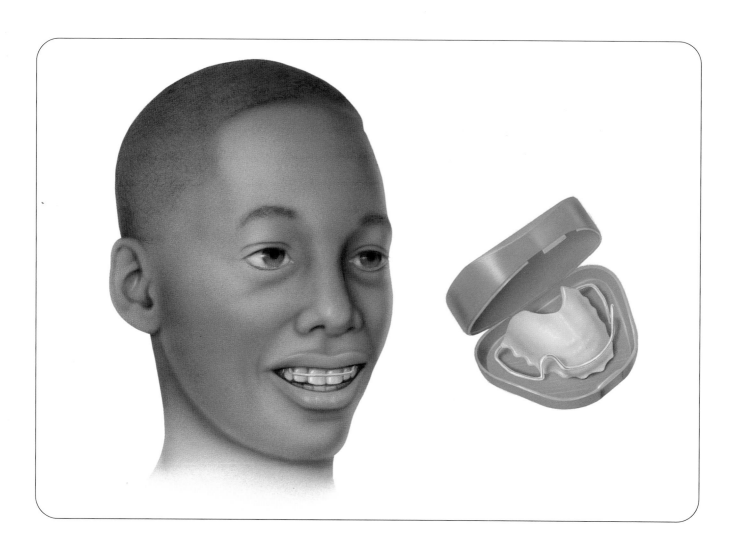

Answers to some commonly asked questions

Do braces hurt?

Not in the same way a skinned knee or a crushed fingernail hurts. Your teeth may feel sore, and eating may be difficult for a day or two after each visit to the dentist. This gradually goes away, and is less after each visit. Often, children's pain reliever will help.

Do spacers hurt?

They may hurt for a few days, but usually children's pain reliever helps.

What if I don't want braces and don't want my teeth to be straight?

You won't starve to death—there are enough foods available today that don't require that much chewing! But you will find that with your crooked teeth and bad bite, it will be much harder to brush and clean your teeth. This could lead to more tooth decay and other problems, such as swollen and bleeding gums, and bad breath. It may also affect the way you talk, swallow, and move your jaw, as well as your smile.

The benefits of being able to chew your food and having straight teeth, a healthy mouth, and an attractive smile would seem to be worth the time and effort.

What are some of the other benefits?

Your mouth will be easier to take care of, your speech may improve, and your teeth will last longer.

What is a retainer and why do I have to wear it?

A retainer is a removable wire and plastic appliance that fits into the top of your mouth. It is worn after your braces have been removed. Even though your teeth are now where they should be, the bone may not be firmly set in place. A retainer holds your teeth in place while the bone hardens.

You may take the retainer out when you eat, but otherwise, you should wear it all the time to make sure your teeth stay straight.

Can I have invisible braces?

"Invisible braces" are braces that are attached to the *insides* of your teeth, or braces that are made of tooth-colored material. This treatment generally lasts longer and costs much more.

Whether invisible braces are right for you also depends on how crooked your teeth are. Sometimes these types of braces aren't strong enough to correct certain problems, and stainless steel appliances are more effective.

How long do I have to wear braces?

That depends on how crooked your teeth are. Your dentist will usually be able to give you an estimate of treatment time before you start, but usually, treatment for a bad bite takes about two or three years.

Why do I have to wear rubber bands?

The rubber bands help move individual teeth or several teeth to improve your bite. You take the rubber bands out yourself when you eat and replace them yourself after you eat. If you need rubber bands, your dentist will give you a supply and show you how to place them.

Will I have to wear a night brace?

This type of appliance is not used all the time, and some dentists don't use it at all. Its main purpose is to hurry the correction of the crooked teeth by applying steady pressure to the teeth. If you do get a night brace, it is very important that you cooperate with your dentist and wear it when you're supposed to.

Can my teeth be straightened with just a retainer or a removable brace?

Some patients' teeth need only minor correction, and in these cases, a retainer or a removable appliance may be used. Your dentist knows best when and where to use these appliances.

How long will I have to wear a retainer?

It depends on your teeth. Your dentist will be able to tell you how long you need to wear a retainer.

How often do I have to go to the dentist for adjustments?

Usually, your dentist will want to adjust your braces about every three to four weeks, maybe more often. Your dentist will tell you how often you should have your braces adjusted.

How often do I have to go to the dentist when my braces come off?

In the beginning, you'll probably have to go to the dentist about every four to six weeks, but the time between visits should gradually extend to every four to six months. The dentist will check your retainer and make sure that your teeth are not moving back to their old positions. Most dentists will want to keep this sort of schedule for a few years.

When I have braces will I have to follow a strict diet?

Not in the regular sense of "diet." Your dentist will ask you to avoid hard foods, sticky or chewy foods, and candy. Eating these things could break or loosen your braces and make it necessary for you to wear them for a longer period. Also, eating sweets increases the chance of cavities during orthodontic treatment.

Will having braces give me cavities?

No, not if you follow your dentist's instructions carefully.

Will it take me an hour to brush my teeth?

No. It will take you a little longer than it has up to now, especially at first, while you learn to clean your teeth and appliance.

Will I have to have teeth pulled?

Sometimes the dentist will need to take out some of your baby teeth to make room for your permanent teeth. Also, if your teeth are extremely crowded, some of your permanent teeth may have to be removed.

If something breaks on my braces, do I have to start treatment all over again?

No, but if you notice that your brackets or bands are loose or broken, you should tell your dentist as soon as you can.

After orthodontic treatment will I need my wisdom teeth removed?

Not all wisdom teeth have enough space to erupt into the mouth after orthodontic treatment. If your dentist thinks that your wisdom teeth will cause problems, he or she may recommend their removal.

Is orthodontic treatment expensive?

Having braces now may eliminate the need for other costly dental and medical care later on, which will save money. Also, if a bad bite is corrected early on, the physical and psychological gains last for a lifetime. So, although the cost may seem high at first, the benefits are spread out over your entire lifetime, making it worthwhile.

If my braces don't work, will I have to have surgery?

Some bad bites are too severe to be treated with braces alone. In these cases, the dentist or orthodontist needs the assistance of another specialist, called an oral surgeon.

Fortunately, such severe cases are rare, but when they occur, the results of braces and surgery combined are often remarkable.